Distribution, publication, and copying in any form are prohibited and subject to damages.

TEN HYPNOSES

Copying, publishing, and sharing with third parties are only permitted with the written consent of the author. Please observe the notes on copyright and usage.

Distribution, publication, and copying in any form are prohibited and subject to damages.

Copying, publishing, and sharing with third parties are only permitted with the written consent of the author. Please observe the notes on copyright and usage.

Distribution, publication, and copying in any form are prohibited and subject to damages.

Ingo Michael Simon

TEN HYPNOSES

21
NAIL BITING

Copying, publishing, and sharing with third parties are only permitted with the written consent of the author. Please observe the notes on copyright and usage.

Distribution, publication, and copying in any form are prohibited and subject to damages.

© 2024 Ingo Michael Simon
All rights reserved.
Independently published
www.ingosimon.com

Important Notes for Urgent Attention:
The contents of this book are based on the practical experiences of the author with hypnosis applications and psychotherapy in a trance state. Although the author has strived for the utmost care, errors or misunderstandings in the presentation cannot be completely excluded. Therapeutic work with people and the application of hypnosis are solely the responsibility of the hypnotist. It cannot be ruled out that parts of this book may be misunderstood or that the application of a presented procedure may cause an undesirable reaction in the client. The author also assumes no co-responsibility if work with a client is carried out with reference to the statements in this book.

The Author:
Ingo Michael Simon studied psychology and education and is a hypnotherapist with practices in southwestern Germany and Switzerland. With the help of hypnosis-supported psychotherapy, he primarily treats people with persistent psychological conditions. His practice focuses on anxiety disorders, pathological compulsions, and psychosomatic illnesses. His therapeutic offerings mainly include classical and modern hypnosis applications and the dreamland therapy he developed himself.

Copying, publishing, and sharing with third parties are only permitted with the written consent of the author. Please observe the notes on copyright and usage.

Notes on Copyright and Usage

Copying, publishing, and sharing with third parties is prohibited and only permitted with the written consent of the author. Please observe the following copyright and usage guidelines.

This work has been carefully crafted and created to the best of the author's knowledge and personal experience. It comprises text templates and application guidelines for professional hypnosis sessions. The author is a licensed psychotherapist with extensive experience in psychotherapy, coaching, and personal training using hypnotic techniques and methods. Nevertheless, the author and the publisher assume no liability for the accuracy of information, instructions, and advice, nor for any typographical errors. The author and publisher accept no responsibility or liability for the application of these texts and recommendations with clients or patients, nor for any potential consequences or unexpected reactions. It is expressly noted that the application of therapeutic and advisory techniques and formulations lies solely and entirely within the responsibility of the practitioner. This also applies to adherence to the boundaries of legally regulated medical and therapeutic practices. The fact that a book containing action proposals is freely available for sale does not imply that its application with clients or patients is permitted for everyone.

Distribution, publication, and copying in any form are prohibited and subject to damages.

Copying, publishing, and sharing with third parties are only permitted with the written consent of the author. Please observe the notes on copyright and usage.

Distribution, publication, and copying in any form are prohibited and subject to damages.

Table of Contents

Introduction	9
Hypnosis 1	11
Hypnosis 2	16
Hypnosis 3	20
Hypnosis 4	25
Hypnosis 5	30
Hypnosis 6	35
Hypnosis 7	40
Hypnosis 8	45
Hypnosis 9	50
Hypnosis 10	55
Overview of All Titles in the Series "Ten Hypnoses"	60

Copying, publishing, and sharing with third parties are only permitted with the written consent of the author. Please observe the notes on copyright and usage.

Distribution, publication, and copying in any form are prohibited and subject to damages.

Copying, publishing, and sharing with third parties are only permitted with the written consent of the author. Please observe the notes on copyright and usage.

Distribution, publication, and copying in any form are prohibited and subject to damages.

Introduction

The series "Ten Hypnoses" is very well known in Germany, Austria, and Switzerland as a collection of texts for therapeutic work and is used by numerous psychotherapeutic practices, doctors, therapists, coaches, and other helping professionals. I am pleased to now be able to offer these texts in other countries as well.

Most therapists have their own methods for inducing and deepening trance as well as for exiting trance. Therefore, I have focused on the main part of the hypnosis. The texts in this book can be integrated as the main part into any hypnosis process.

The texts in this collection use various hypnosis techniques. I will not explain these in detail, as I assume that users have the appropriate training. It is also not necessary to understand the exact structure or functioning of the different parts. The texts can simply be read aloud, and they will have their effect.

Copying, publishing, and sharing with third parties are only permitted with the written consent of the author. Please observe the notes on copyright and usage.

Decide for yourself which text best suits your client or patient at any given time. You can also combine passages from different texts. It is not about using all ten hypnoses in sequence. It is a selection of possibilities.

I want to emphasize that books cannot replace therapy. Psychotherapy or other therapeutic treatments involve much more. A careful diagnosis is the necessary basis for deciding on the use of methods, including whether hypnosis or one of my texts should be used. Even in this case, preparatory discussions, follow-up discussions during the session, and of course, a therapeutic concept for the sequence of sessions and the content approaches are essential parts of therapy. This cannot and should not be achieved with a collection of texts.

In any case, I wish you much success in your work and I am pleased if my text templates can contribute in a small way.

Ingo Michael Simon

Hypnosis 1

Goal Setting and Willpower Strengthening

You have firmly decided to become calmer and more balanced... This one goal is the most important thing you can imagine... To become calmer and leave your fingernails alone... Achieving inner peace to bring about outer peace and leave your fingernails in peace... It's truly astonishing how powerful this single thought becomes... And truly astonishing how strong your will is to make this thought a reality... Peace for you and peace for your fingernails... This is your goal... Your will is your declared will... Your firmly declared will... And nothing and no one can influence your will as strongly as you can yourself... No one can strengthen it as much as you can in this moment... Your will for peace is very strong...

Thought Alignment

You have firmly decided to become calmer and more balanced... Your thoughts are now solely focused on finding peace as quickly as possible... Finding peace and maintaining peace is your goal... And you achieve it faster than you thought... It's quite amazing how your thoughts align to sense signals of peace and allow the feeling of peace to fully exist... Truly astonishing how your thoughts fully align to make peace a reality... This single thought of peace becomes increasingly stable... So stable that it soon turns into a pleasant feeling that you no longer need to think about to find peace... You simply allow it...

Somatic Alignment (Body Suggestion)

At this moment, your body can experience a beautiful state of inner peace... You feel within yourself and can sense this deep relaxation in which you now find yourself... This state invites you to become increasingly tired... As if you want to sleep... As if you want to deeply relax... Now, at this very moment... It's wonderful how well your body follows your will... Your will for deep relaxation... Perhaps you already feel how your body translates this urge for relaxation into deeper relaxation for you... Delving deeper into this beautiful state of inner peace... A peace in which you can deeply sink... And every tension dissolves...

Emotional Alignment (Feeling Suggestion)

Even the deepest tensions are now dissolving... Deep within your feelings, in the realm of your emotions, old tensions are dissolving and freeing you from inner pressure... Thus, it becomes more peaceful within you, and you feel serenity... Deep within you, the feeling of peace exists, now spreading... It's truly astonishing how this peace is already transferring to your fingertips... Exactly this peace frees you from biting and chewing your nails... Exactly this deep relaxation, which is now becoming more pronounced, dissolves all tensions in your body and helps your entire body remain calm and serene... Perhaps you know that emotional relaxation also shows in the relaxation of the body... At this very second...

Behavioral Alignment

You are also now realigning yourself... In this very moment, your body decides to stop chewing your nails... Freed from tension, relaxed and serene as you are now, it becomes a liberation for you to leave your nails alone... You already feel how wonderfully calming it is to leave your fingers completely in peace... Simply enjoying inner peace and serenity, making it increasingly noticeable... You can be proud of yourself for working so intensely on your goal... For continuously aligning yourself now and every coming day to leave your nails alone... Granting peace and serenity to your fingers and teeth by refraining from biting and chewing your nails... A renunciation that becomes freedom... Freedom for you...

Outlook and Vision

You consider how it will be once you have completely stopped biting your nails... You imagine how beautiful and smooth your fingernails can look and that they grow back to a normal length... You also think about how beautiful and relaxing it is once you have entirely stopped biting your nails... How calm it feels and how gentle... Perhaps you have often imagined how restorative it will be once you have stopped biting your nails... Or you are now thinking about it most and most intensely and simply imagining it... And astonishingly, how quickly you transition from imagining to making your thoughts a reality... Never biting your nails again, that will and is your reality...

Summary

The time has come, and there is no other way but to end nail biting now... You have decided it, and you want it... It should now end with nail biting because you no longer need it... All your thoughts have completely aligned with this good goal and help you to truly stop biting your nails now... Your body has understood this feeling of liberation and stores your will in every cell, your will to leave your nails in peace... Deep within your feelings, you sense the desire for peace and relaxation for yourself and your nails... You feel that you succeed today in stopping nail biting... You change your behavior, you leave your nails alone, and you succeed magnificently... You know how wonderful it is to stop biting your nails... Today and continuously stopping...

Reinforcement (Post-hypnotic Suggestion)

And every day, when you look at your fingers and move them, you remember that you have stopped biting your nails... Every movement of your fingers, every contact of your fingers with an object or your body reminds you that you have stopped biting your nails... As soon as your fingernails touch your body, you feel a deep desire to leave your nails in peace and become calmer yourself... Every day...

Hypnosis 2

Goal Setting and Motivation

You have recognized that it's time to take a new path to stop nail biting today... It's truly astonishing how well you succeed in fully focusing on this goal... On the end of nail biting... That's why you have decided to process deeply within what led to the nail biting in the past... It's truly astonishing how well you succeed in now looking deeper and processing the backgrounds of nail biting... Yes, you begin today with the deep and intense processing of all backgrounds and causes of nail biting because that liberates you today... Truly astonishing how well you succeed in exactly that...

Task for the Subconscious

You have recognized that your subconscious can help you, and that's why you have chosen hypnosis to end nail biting and be free... It's truly astonishing how well you succeed in trusting your subconscious now... So you now allow your subconscious to process and release all tensions and conflicts in the depth because this makes you calmer internally and externally, and nail biting disappears on its own... It's truly astonishing how well you succeed in fully trusting your subconscious and feeling that it truly resolves all tensions and conflicts in the depth for you... And nail biting disappears along with it... Yes, you now allow your subconscious to process all tensions and conflicts in the depth and dissolve nail biting along with it... You allow it now... Truly astonishing how well you succeed in exactly that...

Consciousness Control

You have recognized that you reach your goal much faster if you consciously and actively deal with yourself and align your thoughts positively... It's truly astonishing how well you succeed in consciously and actively aligning and steering your thoughts positively... So you now resolve to think and feel consciously and actively... Yes, I process everything inside much faster when I abstain from nail biting, and therefore, this abstinence is also a gain... It's truly astonishing how well you succeed in continuing to trust your subconscious and feeling that it actually processes everything inside even faster with your decision... Yes, you now consciously and actively align your thoughts to fully trust your subconscious and fully support the inner processing... You now consciously and actively align your thoughts... Truly astonishing how well you succeed in exactly that...

Subconscious Processing

Your subconscious has recognized that there was an inner unrest and nervousness that led to nail biting... Your subconscious knows all causes and backgrounds, all unresolved and suppressed feelings that led to this unrest... It's truly astonishing how well your subconscious succeeds in recognizing and understanding these connections... Your subconscious now immediately takes on the task of resolving and processing exactly these causes and backgrounds for you today and then letting them go... Truly astonishing how quickly your subconscious has taken on this task... Truly astonishing how well you work with your subconscious... Yes, your subconscious processes all suppressed feelings in this very moment, allowing them and accepting them, because this dissolves the tension... Dissolving the unrest and you feel relaxation and peace again... Truly astonishing how you already succeed in feeling relaxation and peace again...

Outlook

You have recognized that today is a day of real change, of liberation and a new beginning... Truly astonishing how well you succeed in embracing this change... That's why you continue to trust in the support of your subconscious, which helps you today and every day... Truly astonishing how well you succeed in continuing to trust your subconscious... Yes, you trust your subconscious fully and completely... For the end of nail biting and for new peace and relaxation... Truly astonishing how quickly the end of nail biting is possible...

Hypnosis 3

Anchoring Technique (Perihypnotic Anchor)

An anchor (or trigger) is a stimulus that is supposed to evoke a certain feeling or thought. It is a signal perceived by the client that then initiates an internal process. The set anchor then replaces the suggestion. In everyday life, a client can use an anchor to initiate or establish a desired state without a trance state. Numerous stimuli can be used as anchors/triggers. I work with the following options, which I also use in the series "Ten Hypnoses": body anchors (closing the hand, pressing the thumb ball...), visual anchors (symbols, word cards...), acoustic anchors (signal sounds like phone rings, melodies...), olfactory anchors (essential oils...), haptic anchors (comfort stones, talisman...). I also distinguish between perihypnotic and posthypnotic anchors. Perihypnotic anchors are those that are mainly used during hypnosis, where the therapist sets the anchor and then triggers it repeatedly to complement the suggestions and visualizations. Posthypnotic anchors are mainly set for the time after the session so that the client can help themselves with them.

Preparation of the Anchoring Technique

Today we are working with a special hypnosis technique... A technique that makes it much easier for you to leave nail biting behind and feel good at the same time... To enable this, I will place my hand on your right forearm a few times... Every time you feel my hand on your arm, you know that it is important and that it is part of your hypnosis...

Creating the Desired Emotional State

But first, it's about achieving a beautiful calm state... Because in a state of true inner peace, your fingernails don't matter to you... You feel relaxed now, but you can relax even more and feel how good real inner peace feels... How easy it is to leave your fingers calmly... How easy it is at this moment to simply exhale all tension... Good... very good... You can do it... It works wonderfully... You just let go... You feel a deep and pleasant peace within you... And you have the desire to delve even deeper into this beautiful state of inner peace... Very deep...

Setting the Anchor

Nail biting is like holding onto your fingernails, biting into them... But you want to let go of your nails, and that happens through inner peace and serenity... At this moment, you feel... [hand placed]... peace and serenity... [hand removed]... Deep within you, you can... [hand placed]... feel peace and serenity... [hand removed]... So you have no urge to bite your nails, absolutely none, because you feel... [hand placed]... peace and serenity... [hand removed]... Perhaps you think about how nice it would be to always feel this... [hand placed]... peace and serenity... [hand removed]... And perhaps that is possible... Because somewhere inside you, even in stressful times, there is a bit of... [hand placed]... peace and serenity... [hand removed]... that you can find...

[By now, the therapist's hand has become the anchor for the feeling of "peace and serenity." Each further touch emphasizes this feeling. The client can thus deal with nail biting and receive a constant impulse of peace. This breaks the connection between stress and nail biting. The client will not start nail biting in a state of calm.]

Using the Anchor

You think again about... [hand placed]... nail biting... [hand removed]... Often you didn't notice that you were doing it... Then again, you noticed and always tried to stop... Sometimes it works... [hand placed]... to just stop and still feel good... [hand removed]... You now know that... [hand placed]... nail biting was a kind of stress reaction... or a release of stress... [hand removed]... You don't need that now, because you can... [hand placed]... avoid stress... [hand removed]... You can... [hand placed]... prevent inner stress overload... [hand removed]... by always aiming for a relaxed state... Now, at this moment, you feel no stress, even though you are thinking about... [hand placed]... your fingernails... [hand removed]... They are very short, but perhaps you have the desire to let them grow a little longer... That works best when you succeed in always finding peace again... [hand placed]... finding peace after excitement... Also in conflict, finding as much peace as possible... In disputes or worries, at least finding some peace... [hand removed]...

Reinforcement (Post-hypnotic Suggestion)

Good... You have already learned everything you need to know and can do to stop biting your nails for good and feel good about it... Just as good as now... Because now you are not biting your nails and feel good... It works every day exactly like this because you succeed in releasing your stress... letting go of your fear... Whatever burdens you, let it go... You do it exactly as I did today... As soon as you notice inner unrest, you grab one arm with the other hand and immediately feel inner peace... and let go... With a little pressure on the arm, you can intensify the effect even more... [hand placed again and pressing firmly but not too hard]... becoming even calmer... Just like this... Exactly like this...

Hypnosis 4

Anchoring Technique (Post-hypnotic Anchor)

An anchor (or trigger) is a stimulus that is supposed to evoke a certain feeling or thought. It is a signal perceived by the client that then initiates an internal process. The set anchor then replaces the suggestion. In everyday life, a client can use an anchor to initiate or establish a desired state without a trance state. Numerous stimuli can be used as anchors/triggers. I work with the following options, which I also use in the series "Ten Hypnoses": body anchors (closing the hand, pressing the thumb ball...), visual anchors (symbols, word cards...), acoustic anchors (signal sounds like phone rings, melodies...), olfactory anchors (essential oils...), haptic anchors (comfort stones, talisman...). I also distinguish between perihypnotic and posthypnotic anchors. Perihypnotic anchors are those that are mainly used during hypnosis, where the therapist sets the anchor and then triggers it repeatedly to complement the suggestions and visualizations. Posthypnotic anchors are mainly set for the time after the session so that the client can help themselves with them.

Preparation of the Anchoring Technique

Today we are working with a special hypnosis technique... A technique that makes it much easier for you to leave nail biting behind and feel good at the same time... To enable this, I help you set up an anchor... You can then use the anchor anytime and anywhere to quickly reach a state of calmness, so you don't even think about nail biting... Closing your right hand into a loose fist will be your anchor... But until we set it up, you can relax...

Creating the Desired Emotional State

First, it's about reaching a deep state of inner peace... Because in a state of true inner peace, you don't even think about biting your nails... Peace and stress don't coexist... If you feel inner peace, even a little, stress automatically dissipates... You feel very relaxed at this moment, you are not biting your nails because you are relaxed... Because you feel inner peace... But you can relax even more and feel how good real inner peace feels... How easy it is to leave your fingers calmly... How easy it is at this moment to simply let go of all tension that might still be there and feel peace... Good... You are doing it right... You are doing it exactly right... It works wonderfully... You just let go... You feel a deep and pleasant peace within you... And you have the desire to delve even deeper into this beautiful state of inner peace... Very deep... You remember a time or an event of deep peace... Perhaps a lovely nap or a deep meditation... A calm evening watching TV or a wonderful massage that helped you relax... And as you remember, you actually relax even deeper... And enter a state of deep and very pleasant inner peace...

Setting the Anchor

We will now anchor this state of deep and pleasant peace together... We will establish it in your body so that you can find it again whenever you need it... Two things are important for this... First, focusing on the feeling of peace to feel it intensely now... Second, paying attention and mindfulness to your hands and fingers to feel them in this peace as well... Then direct your attention to your right hand and close it into a fist as soon as you feel you cannot relax any deeper... Close your right hand into a loose fist...

[Wait until the client closes their fist. If it doesn't happen, which is rare, help with suggestions... You are already more deeply relaxed than you might think... You can close your fist now, as this will help you relax even more... Close your hand into a fist now...]

Good, now feel the relaxation even more intensely... Your body has already learned that closing your right hand into a fist is a signal for immediate relaxation... And if you want to relax even more deeply, squeeze your fist a little tighter... Just squeeze your fist tighter and come to rest... Good... Very good... Your anchor works... Now release the pressure and slowly open your fist... Very slowly, as this will allow you to feel that the peace remains... When your anchor is triggered, like a switch you press, your entire body, your entire being, enters a state of pleasant peace and stays there as long as possible... Open your hand slowly and relax your fingers... You can feel that the inner peace remains... And your fingernails no longer matter... You have no urge to bite them, none at all... None at all... Your fingers relax with you...

Reinforcement (Post-hypnotic Suggestion)

Good... You have already internalized everything you need to stop biting your nails for good and feel truly calm and good... Just as you experienced now... Because now you are not biting your nails and now you are not interested in your fingernails at all... This can succeed every day exactly like today... Because you succeed in letting go of everything that could burden you... You do it exactly like today... As soon as you think or feel that inner unrest might arise, direct your attention to your right hand and close it slowly into a fist to easily refrain from biting your nails... Then you feel how you become calmer inside, significantly calmer... And if you want to become even calmer, just squeeze the fist tighter... Exactly as you succeeded today... Exactly like today...

Hypnosis 5

Goal Setting and Preparation

You want to stop biting your nails; you want to end it once and for all... You have already tried, but it hasn't worked quite right... But you have the firm will to leave your fingernails alone in the future... You know that nail biting had a function, so it made sense to nibble on them... You thought it was a signal of stress and inner tension, and perhaps that was a large part of it... So if you can relax... sustainably relax, you don't need nail biting as much... But then you still haven't quite stopped... Because there is something you haven't seen yet... Something that often prompted you to bite your nails... Today you are on the path to finding this exact function and then dissolving it...

Perspective Shift

Imagine you were a tiger... And the people you have conflicts with or are afraid of are also powerful tigers... Imagine powerful people as mighty, large tigers... Superiors maybe, or teachers... People who can test and evaluate you... Individuals who are faster or stronger in confrontation than you... Imagine all of them as tigers... These tigers have scared you... Perhaps you often felt uncertainty or even fear of them... Or you had a feeling of tension inside, a queasy feeling in your stomach... And yet, it was actually a certain fear... From this sometimes came anger... You might have often wanted to pound your fists on the table... Or drum on it... You might have wanted to extend your tiger claws and defend yourself... Like a tiger that can fend off attacks and attackers with its long and strong claws... But you trimmed your claws... You chewed your claws to be less dangerous... To be reserved... Without claws, you couldn't defend yourself, so the entire pressure remained inside you... You imagine the many tigers in your life... Perhaps they aren't so many... Perhaps only a few who were particularly powerful or were when you learned to trim your inner claws... And to bite your fingernails...

Reevaluating Own Experiences

Now you dive back into your memories and a situation comes to mind where you intensely chewed your nails... Imagine the situation again and imagine you had tiger paws instead of hands... And now clearly imagine how you chewed your tiger claws in this situation... Perhaps you could have also defended yourself against what really bothered or strained you... Especially if they were inner things... Memories or feelings you fought with... Because, strictly speaking, you didn't fight, you prevented yourself from fighting... Without claws, no tiger can fight... Without claws, no tiger can defend itself... Remember this situation and stand beside yourself... Watch yourself chewing your tiger claws... How you made yourself a tiger without claws... Perhaps you can already see that you often would have preferred to defend yourself rather than chew your nails... Imagine many tigers standing before you, with sharp claws, and you chew and chew your claws to be a very nice tiger... Hoping to be spared... There they stand, the tigers of insults... Tigers of fear... Tigers of despair... Tigers of helplessness... And such tigers that only you know... Their claws remain dangerous...

Action Shift

Now, in your imagination, before your inner eye, you change this... Imagine you stop chewing your claws and nails... And imagine them growing back... With each breath, your tiger claws now grow... In your inner images, this is possible; it goes very quickly... And deep inside, it happens just as quickly... Your fingernails are just an outer reflection of what happened deep inside... So in your inner images, they also grow back quickly as soon as you stop trimming your inner claws... As soon as you allow your claws... Claws of anger... Claws of rage... Claws of freedom that help you be yourself... You now see before your inner eye how you extend your claws... Like a cat that had only retracted its claws and was gentle, you now extend your tiger claws again... And at the same time, you see how the tigers become more cautious... Cautious tigers of insults... Cautious tigers of fear... Cautious tigers of despair... Cautious tigers of helplessness... And such cautious tigers that only you know... The inner tigers that have threatened you so often become gentler, and you gain strength...

Reinforcement (Post-hypnotic Suggestion)

You now feel inner peace and relaxation... You feel and know that you can fend off the tigers inside you... You feel and know that you can extend your claws again and again... And every time you feel the urge to bite your nails, you feel the much stronger urge to extend your claws and defend yourself... That's why you refrain from biting your nails... To keep your claws intact... Just like today in your imagination, you succeed every day in your waking life...

Hypnosis 6

Goal Setting and Preparation

You have decided to stop biting your nails; you want to end it for good... You have tried it a few times already, but then you started again, perhaps without noticing it... But you have the strong will to leave your fingernails alone in the future... You know that nail biting wasn't an accident but had meaning, so it was logical to do it in certain situations... You thought it was just too much stress, or you couldn't quite understand why you bit your nails... If you can relax... really deeply relax, you don't need nail biting... Just like now... But it wasn't so easy to compete with habitual nail biting using relaxation... Because there were feelings and moods that repeatedly prompted you to bite your nails... Feelings that you haven't seen and haven't freed yet... So you are on the path to discovering these exact feelings and then letting them rise and feel them... And then also freeing them so they can't build up pressure anymore...

Perspective Shift

Perhaps you thought you could feel your emotions well... Because you often felt insecure or could feel this pressure inside you... This tension that discharged by biting your nails... And yet there is more... There are suppressed feelings and moods... Perhaps injuries... Or offenses inside you... Perhaps you also feel a deep anger and never allowed yourself to express or release your rage... Many feelings can be within you, deep inside, waiting to be freed because every freed feeling reduces inner pressure as soon as it is seen... Imagine your feelings are like balloons... And each balloon represents a feeling... And because feelings want to be released, these balloons are filled with a very light gas... With helium... They would rise immediately, fly into the sky and be very light if they weren't held back... But today it's about the deep feelings you have often suppressed, probably had to suppress, because you couldn't deal with them otherwise... So this huge bunch of balloons is tied to an iron railing... Imagine how many gas balloons are tied to an iron railing, pulling upwards to free themselves... They pull and dance in the wind but can't get loose yet...

Reevaluating Own Experiences

Now imagine how it was when you bit your nails... Deep inside, these balloons were there, which you still imagine before your inner eye... They pulled and danced, trying to come to the surface because they wanted to be seen and felt... But something in you didn't allow it... You bit your nails... You now see a picture of what it would be like if you were standing at the iron railing with the many dancing balloons, biting your nails... You can't free the balloons now because you would need to untie the knots holding them... You would need your fingernails, which you are biting in your inner imagination now... Now remember a particular feeling you have long wanted to release, whatever it may be... This feeling has also been tied to the iron railing for years... Perhaps because you thought it was a bad or inappropriate feeling... But such a thing doesn't exist... Actions can be bad, but not feelings...

Action Shift

Images before our inner eye are always a reflection of what is possible deep in our feelings... And today, it is possible to free a large part of your suppressed feelings... To finally let them rise so they can be free and light... So now imagine untying the strings holding the balloons and freeing the balloons of feelings... One by one, you untie them... And immediately the balloons of feelings rise... They fly upwards into the sky, and you watch them... [Ensure the client exhales while you say "pressure releases"]... The balloons of freed feelings float lightly upwards... Rising higher and higher... And the pressure releases... Watch them... All freed balloons... All freed feelings... And the pressure releases... Balloons of disappointment fly high... And the pressure releases... Balloons of anger fly high... And the pressure releases... Balloons of fear fly high... And the pressure releases... All feelings rise like balloons... All feelings rise like balloons... And the pressure releases... And as soon as they have been sufficiently seen, they burst in the wind...

Reinforcement (Post-hypnotic Suggestion)

You imagine that it can be good to let your own feelings rise like untethered gas balloons every day, which want to go upwards... So pressure can release every day because only suppressed feelings build pressure, freed feelings always relieve... So your body adjusts to the fact that leaving your fingernails alone is a signal for you to release all balloons of suppressed feelings... If you have the impulse to bite your nails and refrain from doing so, the balloons of your feelings are freed deep inside and rise... Are seen by you and felt by you and burst in the wind... Just like today... Exactly like today...

Hypnosis 7

Goal Setting and Preparation

You often bite your nails... You are about to change that, but it's not just about stopping it... Of course, it's pleasant and good if you stop biting your nails because it bothers you, and this disturbance will then be over... At the same time, there is a reason for biting and nibbling on your nails... Many reasons, perhaps, if you look at individual situations and events that lead to nail biting the fastest... But only one reason if we look at the principle behind it... If you succeed in understanding nail biting as a substitute action, as an abreaction of tension that you couldn't control quickly otherwise, it can succeed very quickly to change this reaction... To react differently to stress or fear... To deal differently and newly with tensions... Often it was so that you didn't

even really notice that you were internally tense... You only noticed it because you suddenly started biting your nails... So if you can succeed in feeling internal tension coming up faster, you can also react appropriately and leave your fingers in peace... Then you don't need to bite your nails... You just have to notice in time that tension is coming up to be able to let it go or handle it appropriately...

Somato-emotional Change

Here your body feeling helps you... Because internal tension shows in a certain restlessness in your fingertips and in your lower jaw... On the tips of your teeth... Teeth and fingertips then react to it, and it leads to nail biting... Maybe it has been clear to you for a long time that it was the felt restlessness in fingertips and teeth that caused it... Or it is only now becoming clear to you that it was so... Every body has its peculiarities, and in our body, what we think and feel always shows... If we feel tension from stress, time pressure, performance pressure, or fear, this tension bites into our body somewhere... For you, in the fingertips and teeth... If it succeeds to have an image in your mind instead of body tension, nail biting becomes unnecessary...

So now direct your mindfulness to your teeth... Leave the fingernails unnoticed for now, but concentrate on your teeth, on the tooth tips... Because that's where what makes you so restless sits... Then remember the last situation where you strongly bit your nails... Imagine once again how it was and how it felt in your teeth... Maybe you also feel tension in the tooth tips now or everything feels very loose and calm because you can't access this feeling yet... Concentrate on your teeth and feel how the tension becomes noticeable there... But you succeed wonderfully in enduring it now... Then pay attention to your fingertips, because that feeling of tension sits there too... Concentrate on your fingertips... But you can endure that well today too... You are doing it very well... Now imagine that what has put you under so much pressure is now loosening from your fingertips and teeth and slowly wandering as a feeling into your head... The stress sitting in fingers and teeth now flows into your thoughts... Step by step, the pressure loosens from fingers and teeth and gently flows through your body to your head... Very gently... Because it is just a feeling... And feelings never harm... Even strenuous or painful feelings do not harm but help us understand ourselves better... All feelings from fingertips and teeth now gently flow to your thoughts... And in your head, a picture of what really put you under so much pressure emerges... Now, a picture of what made you so restless during the last nail biting emerges... And the tension in the teeth disappears at this very moment... Maybe you already have this picture clearly before your inner eye... Or you can perceive it more clearly a bit later... But everything that sat in fingertips and teeth now flows into your thoughts and can be perceived by you as an image... Or as a word... As a thought... You now know what really put you under so much pressure... You now feel this feeling that no longer sits in fingers and teeth but in your consciousness... Your body learns to always do it like this for you... Unpleasant or hard-to-grasp feelings no longer get pushed into your fingertips and teeth but get brought as images and perceptible feelings into your thoughts... Your fingernails give up all feelings arriving there immediately to your thoughts... Also, your teeth push all feelings arriving there immediately back into your thoughts so you can feel what it's really about... So you can react appropriately to burdens... And nail biting becomes the past... The completed past...

Reinforcement (Post-hypnotic Suggestion)

And if the feeling of wanting to bite your nails comes up again or if it just happens in the hustle of everyday life, then simply close your eyes briefly, concentrate briefly on your fingertips, and then on your teeth, and ask your body what sits there... Immediately, your body will provide you an answer by sending exactly the feelings sitting in fingertips and teeth into your thoughts... Just like today... Every day, exactly like today...

Hypnosis 8

Ideomotor phenomenon describes the occurrence that our body follows our feelings and thoughts with movements. In everyday life, this following is shown as body posture, muscle tension, and movement patterns of a person, which naturally change with the mood and thoughts. In trance, ideomotor signals can be used to receive information that the client cannot actively communicate. The subconscious can, for example, answer questions with an agreed finger signal. Of course, ideomotor reactions can also be used suggestively, for example, with arm levitations and catalepsies. Such an approach, which I also use in the following text, strengthens trust in hypnosis and in one's own ability to change, thereby promoting therapy.

Goal Setting and Preparation

You want to stop biting your nails... You have already tried, but now you want it to finally succeed... For this, we use your subconscious's ability to communicate with us through body signals... Your subconscious can send signals with the help of your body reactions and show you what changes are possible... Our subconscious does this constantly; we just aren't always open to receiving these signals or don't understand them correctly... Today that is different because I help you perceive your subconscious's signals clearly... You have already dealt with nail biting, understood that it was a form of stress relief... A spontaneous and often unconscious reaction to reduce stress... It happened so quickly that you only noticed it when you already felt the fingernails between your teeth... Now you succeed in feeling inner unrest and stress faster and then reacting differently, reacting earlier, even before nail biting starts, counteracting stress... Now your body must leave this old routine and stop nail biting... Your subconscious can do that for you and show you that it has actually done it... So let's get started...

Inducing Catalepsy

Now concentrate on your desire to stop nail biting... And give your subconscious the task to support you in this... So that you absolutely and completely succeed in stopping nail biting... First, imagine your fingers getting longer... Imagine it for both hands, just like that... As a fantasy... Imagine your fingers getting longer and longer... They stretch longer and grow... It's as if the fingers become very long... Thirty centimeters long... And even longer... Your fingers stretch and grow down to your feet... And then further... Imagine you are standing next to yourself and can observe it... Your fingers getting longer and longer... They are already two meters long... Too long to chew and nibble on... You have very long fingers... And they keep growing longer... Five meters long... Ten meters long... They drill through the wall and grow across the city... And every thought of nail biting makes your fingers even longer now... And every attempt to bend or move your fingers immediately makes them longer... Immediately longer... Good... Your subconscious shows you that it can help you prevent nail biting... Here today in trance and then also in your waking everyday life... Every attempt to move your fingers now makes them longer... Longer and firmer... Every single attempt to move your fingers now makes them longer... Longer and firmer... Good...

Ideomotor Command

You stop nail biting... It has become impossible... It doesn't work now... You would have to move your fingers to do so, but that no longer works because they immediately grow longer... Try it... Move your fingers, which now get longer... Once more... Move your fingers, which now get longer... It no longer works... It's impossible to bite your nails now because your subconscious no longer wants it... Every time you try to move your fingers to bite your nails, they get longer... Try it once more... Once more... Good... Your subconscious can do it... You can do it...

[If the client can still bend their fingers, suggest again several times that they become longer and firmer. Observe the fingers while doing so. You can observe the active stretching with the suggestion "become longer." Then have the client try to move their fingers again. It will not work if you quickly enough say the suggestion "... become longer." Also, try instructing the client simply to move their fingers. If the catalepsy is stable, this will no longer work.]

Resolving Catalepsy

Your subconscious can block nail biting... But it can also give you freedom and mobility... Imagine your fingers getting shorter again... Completely flexible and soft, like rubber... Your fingers getting shorter again... And completely normally flexible... At this moment, your fingers become completely flexible and completely normal again... Your subconscious does this for you... And relaxes your fingers... They are completely loose... As loose as rubber... Now move your fingers naturally and check that it is true... You can move your fingers... Good...

[Always make sure the client has control of their fingers again and can move them. Let them actively try. If it doesn't work, help with further suggestions... Your fingers are totally relaxed, completely loose. Your fingers are very, very loose...]

Reinforcement (Post-hypnotic Suggestion)

Your subconscious was able to stop you from biting your nails today... It can do this every day... Because every time you want to start biting your nails, your subconscious can stretch your fingers and show you that you no longer need to bite them... Every time you are tempted, your subconscious reacts by stretching your fingers and you feel this impulse reminding you that you don't need to bite your nails anymore... Just like today... Exactly like here and today...

Hypnosis 9

Arriving in the Land of Dreams

Imagination often seems to contradict reality... Yet sometimes both are very close to each other... Then imagination can easily become truth... Deep in our thoughts and feelings... And then also in the exterior of our lives... There is a special place where the imaginations that can all become truth arise... It is a place only you can go to because it lies somewhere deep in your feelings...

The land of your dreams... You reach it with the power of your thoughts and your creativity... You just imagine you can slip out of yourself with one of the next breaths... Overcome the boundaries of your body to be completely free... To go on a journey as a free spirit... A journey to the land of dreams, which is vast... As infinitely large as the world of your feelings... You exhale and go to the land of dreams...

Confrontation, Clarification, and Creative Realignment

You stand on a wide path that looks like an old gray road... The asphalt is broken and the road is bumpy and uneven... As bumpy as your life sometimes was... As uneven and brittle as you sometimes feel deep inside... In the land of dreams, the color gray stands for all the bad and wrong things in your life... For everything you have suffered from or are suffering from... Also for the stress and fear that repeatedly led to your nail biting... You continue walking this bumpy path because it too will lead you to a good goal, which in the land of dreams is always you... In the infinite vastness and size of the land, you can also find new paths, a new way to deal with yourself... [White]... Your path leads through a field of flowers made up of thousands of white flowers, daisies, or your favorite white flower... And the path under your feet also turns white... The color white shows you in the land of dreams that there is always hope and always possibilities to clear up the grayness of life... To dissolve the gray shadows of the past and be free again... Free from fear and stress, free from compulsion and the feeling of being small... So you succeed in the imagination of the color white to believe that there is change, that you can stand strong without biting your nails... [Light Blue]... Then you look up to the sky, seeing the bright blue sky of the dream land... A radiant blue sky, so open and wide... The color light blue shows you in the land of dreams that the infinite vastness of life is open to you again once you succeed in lovingly letting go of the past because you can no longer change the past... Letting go of the desire for retribution and revenge or for making up for everything you have suffered... This also allows you to accept the present and act completely in the present... To start anew every day and do everything differently that you can and want to do differently... [Ochre/Gold Yellow]... Your path leads you to a wheat field... The color of the wheat, the ochre that in its shining form becomes a beautiful golden yellow, is the color of learning, recognizing, and understanding... You have already learned and recognized so much in your life, but here in the land of dreams, it is always about finding and understanding your own feelings... The feelings behind the nervousness, the feelings that really belong to you, not what was trained... The color gold yellow helps you feel your true feelings... [Red]... You continue walking, step by step, and come to a field of roses... A huge field full of red roses, which here in the land of dreams have no thorns... Often the thorns of life have driven you forward, but here it is different... Here the roses proclaim love... Especially self-love that allows you to find yourself good, to like yourself, to love yourself... The red roses allow you to love yourself as you are, exactly as you are... In the land of dreams and in your waking everyday life... Whether you bite your nails or not... Love yourself as you are... [Silver]... Then you come to a silver archway and as you pass under the arch, you are bathed in silver light... Like small silver stars raining down on you and settling on your body... Silver is in the land of dreams the color of constructive future... The truth that can be when the right time comes... And perhaps this time is now, this very second, and the color silver helps you to end nail biting because you no longer need it in a constructive and new future... [Gold]... Then you discover a small spring from which golden water gushes... Gold is the color of the greatest strength within you, the color of creative power... This power was given to you with your birth, with your life... Now, in the land of dreams, you can use it again, can feel your own strength and power because you are part of creation...

Mindfulness and Self-loyalty

Then you come to a meadow on a high plateau... You had not noticed until now that you were so high up, but from here you can overlook the entire land of dreams, can recognize and view everything... The land of dreams is waiting to be discovered and explored by you... To find your new path without nail biting, because when you find your own feelings, you feel so free that you never need it again... Then you lie down comfortably, and it becomes clear to you that this special world truly exists... Not only in your imagination but deep inside you, the land of dreams exists... It has always been there... I'm just telling you about it...

Hypnosis 10

Arriving in the Land of Dreams

Imagination often seems to contradict reality... Yet sometimes both are very close to each other... Then imagination can easily become truth... Deep in our thoughts and feelings... And then also in the exterior of our lives... There is a special place where the imaginations that can all become truth arise... It is a place only you can go to because it lies somewhere deep in your feelings... The land of your dreams... You reach it with the power of your thoughts and your creativity... You just imagine you can slip out of yourself with one of the next breaths... Overcome the boundaries of your body to be completely free... To go on a journey as a free spirit... A journey to the land of dreams, which is vast... As infinitely large as the world of your feelings... You exhale and go to the land of dreams...

Confrontation, Clarification, and Creative Realignment

You stand on a huge meadow, directly under an old tree... In the shade of the tree, you feel safe... But you are interested in the land of dreams and look out from under the branches of the tree... You can look infinitely far into the distance... The land of dreams looks like you imagine a beautiful land because beyond the large meadow, there is everything you can think of... Mountains and valleys... Rivers and lakes... Blooming plants and trees with ripe fruits... You take a few steps over the meadow and look up at the sky... The weather is just as you like it best... Then you look at the old tree... You walk around it... It looks as if many storm fronts have swept over it... The tips of many branches are broken because whenever it became really stormy, too much tension acted on the branches... The trunk of the tree is thick and firm; it will not bend... This tree can withstand a lot... But on the outside, at the ends of the branches, it cracks here and there in the storm... The tree stands alone on a very large meadow... As beautiful and diverse as the land of dreams may be, this tree stands here alone in the wind... You think about how you can protect its branches... So that they don't wear out at the ends... You look over the meadow and discover a sign in the middle of this meadow... You walk to the sign and can read the inscription... It says "Meadow of the One Tree" and below that is your name... It is as if you yourself once decided that this tree should stand alone in the wind... But you feel that this can't be... Then you think about how you often feel this inner tension and then nibble on your nails to somehow become calmer... Perhaps you once learned to be quiet and to deal with the inner pressure on your own... Because there was no one to help you release your tension or was willing to... You look up at the sky, which turns ochre and becomes a huge screen... On this screen, you suddenly see pictures and scenes from your childhood... You see again, like in a film, how it was in the past... When you had inner pressure and couldn't release it... Perhaps because it was forbidden... Or because you were afraid... Or for another reason you can now recognize in the old pictures... But even if you don't know why it happened that you started biting your nails to relieve tension, that's completely okay... Because it only matters to be here in the land of dreams now, because here you understand that it couldn't have been different back then... Somehow you had to deal with the pressure... Somehow you have to deal with it until today... Nail biting was a solution for a long time... But you don't need this solution now because you know you don't stand alone in the wind like the tree on the meadow... Because deep inside, you know how to reduce stress... You have also long since learned not to swallow things or cling to them... Today you learn from these old images of your childhood how to express your feelings of tension, to give them a way, so that the inner storm of feelings doesn't come up anymore... You learn it by yourself, need to do nothing for it... You just have to be there... Let the images of the dreamland work, that is already enough... You look up at the sky and now see pictures and scenes from your adult life... Can recognize situations in which you particularly strongly nibbled on your nails... But then you look down again... Search the ground and find a leather pouch... You take it in your hand and open it... In the pouch is a special seed... Golden grains are in the pouch, and each little golden grain stands for one of your unspoken feelings... You think back and realize that you have often held back your moods and feelings... Whether anger or rage... Anger and worry... Disappointment and frustration... Fear or anxiety... You have often held them back and then felt tension that you tried to reduce by biting your nails... Here in the land of dreams, you now release these unspoken feelings... You walk over the meadow and spread the golden grains of your feelings like seeds from the pouch, distributing your feelings all over the meadow... And you feel how you become freer and calmer... You distribute the seeds everywhere on the meadow until you are back under the old tree and get tired... Then you sit down, and it starts to rain... Warm rain falls from the bright blue sky, and everywhere a golden seed lies, a new silver tree grows before your eyes like in a time-lapse... You watch as many silver trees grow and rise in the land of dreams... Until finally, the old tree is surrounded by many protective trees... So protected that the ends of the branches no longer break in the wind... Because the storm no longer comes up, it loses itself in the growing trees of feelings, in the land of dreams...

Mindfulness and Self-loyalty

You close your eyes and rest... You dream a beautiful dream of never biting your nails again because you no longer need it... And this dream becomes truth... Today already... Or tomorrow... Or every day of your further life a bit more... Then you think about the fact that the land of dreams is deep inside you... It has always been there... I'm just telling you about it...

Distribution, publication, and copying in any form are prohibited and subject to damages.

Copying, publishing, and sharing with third parties are only permitted with the written consent of the author. Please observe the notes on copyright and usage.

Overview of All Titles in the Series "Ten Hypnoses"

Volume 1: Smoking Cessation
Volume 2: Anxiety and Restlessness
Volume 3: Burnout
Volume 4: Reducing Overweight
Volume 5: Coping with the Past
Volume 6: Suicidal Thoughts and Attempts
Volume 7: Psycho-Oncology
Volume 8: Obsessions and Tics
Volume 9: Self-Confidence and Decision-Making
Volume 10: Grief Work
Volume 11: Psychosomatics
Volume 12: Chronic Pain
Volume 13: Depressive Thoughts
Volume 14: Panic Attacks
Volume 15: Domestic Violence, Victim Support
Volume 16: Post-Traumatic Stress
Volume 17: Exam Anxiety and Stage Fright
Volume 18: Anti-Violence Training, Offender Support
Volume 19: Addiction Tendencies
Volume 20: Social Phobia and Fear of Contact
Volume 21: Nail Biting
Volume 22: Self-Awareness and Self-Love
Volume 23: Teeth Grinding and Night Clenching
Volume 24: Feelings of Guilt
Volume 25: Fear in Crowds
Volume 26: Fear of Flying, Aviophobia
Volume 27: Fear in Enclosed Spaces, Claustrophobia
Volume 28: Tinnitus, Ear Noises
Volume 29: Fear of Heights
Volume 30: Neurodermatitis

Copying, publishing, and sharing with third parties are only permitted with the written consent of the author. Please observe the notes on copyright and usage.

Volume 31: Finding Inner Balance
Volume 32: Overcoming Loneliness
Volume 33: Fear of Illness, Hypochondria
Volume 34: Anticipatory Anxiety, Fear of Fear
Volume 35: Jealousy in Relationships
Volume 36: Driving Anxiety
Volume 37: New Start after Separation
Volume 38: Fear of Injections
Volume 39: Heart Anxiety Neurosis
Volume 40: Overcoming Resentment and Anger
Volume 41: Resolving Blockages and Positive Thinking
Volume 42: Stress Reduction, Stress Management
Volume 43: Body Relaxation
Volume 44: Deep Relaxation
Volume 45: Fear of the Dark
Volume 46: Falling Asleep and Staying Asleep
Volume 47: Compulsive Buying
Volume 48: Restless Legs Syndrome
Volume 49: Bulimia
Volume 50: Anorexia
Volume 51: Overcoming Nightmares
Volume 52: Imagined Deformity
Volume 53: Overcoming Distrust, Finding Trust
Volume 54: Processing Failures
Volume 55: Humiliation, Emotional Hurt
Volume 56: Distressing Compassion, Vicarious Suffering
Volume 57: Self-Forgiveness
Volume 58: Self-Awareness, Self-Confidence
Volume 59: Saying No
Volume 60: Assertiveness
Volume 61: Setting Boundaries and Self-Assertion
Volume 62: Decision-Making Ability

Volume 63: Success Orientation
Volume 64: Ruminating, Circular Thinking
Volume 65: Accepting Pregnancy
Volume 66: Birth Preparation
Volume 67: Spiritual Opening
Volume 68: Joy of Life and Inner Lightness
Volume 69: Patience and Inner Peace
Volume 70: Fibromyalgia and Rheumatism
Volume 71: Irritable Bowel Syndrome, Crohn's Disease
Volume 72: Fear of Nausea, Emetophobia
Volume 73: Stuttering and Cluttering, Speech Flow Disorders
Volume 74: Concentration and Knowledge Anchoring
Volume 75: Vitality and Spontaneity
Volume 76: Searching for Meaning and Finding Goals
Volume 77: Life Crises, Life Events
Volume 78: Workaholism, Goal Obsession
Volume 79: Helper Syndrome, Helpless Helpers
Volume 80: Medication Abuse
Volume 81: Gambling Addiction
Volume 82: Internet Addiction, Smartphone Addiction
Volume 83: Hoarding Disorder, Compulsive Collecting
Volume 84: Conspiracy Thoughts, Overvalued Ideas
Volume 85: Fear of Operations and Treatments
Volume 86: Fear of Aging
Volume 87: Travel Anxiety
Volume 88: Anxiety When Urinating, Paruresis
Volume 89: Fear of Intimacy and Togetherness
Volume 90: Fear of Blushing
Volume 91: Coming Out in Homosexuality
Volume 92: Charisma Training
Volume 93: Migraines and Chronic Headaches
Volume 94: Overcoming Allergies, Bronchial Asthma

Volume 95: Normalizing Blood Pressure
Volume 96: Compulsive Perfectionism
Volume 97: Sports Hypnosis, Motivation
Volume 98: Sports Hypnosis, Performance Enhancement
Volume 99: Determination and Focus
Volume 100: Encountering the Inner Child
Volume 101: Cravings, Binge Eating
Volume 102: Stimulating Metabolism
Volume 103: Bipolar Mood Swings
Volume 104: Borderline, Identity Crises
Volume 105: Hypomania, Euphoria, Mania
Volume 106: Restlessness, Agitation
Volume 107: Nervous Breakdown
Volume 108: Adjustment Disorders
Volume 109: Self-Alienation, Depersonalization
Volume 110: Ending Self-Pity
Volume 111: Primary Gain of Illness
Volume 112: Secondary Gain of Illness
Volume 113: Bullying, Victim Support
Volume 114: Letting Go of Envy and Jealousy
Volume 115: Fear of Spiders, Arachnophobia
Volume 116: Fear of Dogs or Cats
Volume 117: Fear of Strangers, Xenophobia
Volume 118: Excessive Worries, Generalized Anxiety
Volume 119: Strengthening Sense of Responsibility
Volume 120: Unrequited Love, Heartache
Volume 121: Work-Life Balance
Volume 122: Letting Go of Unattainable Goals
Volume 123: Allowing and Accepting Help
Volume 124: Letting Go of Adult Children
Volume 125: Tourette Syndrome
Volume 126: Life Changes and New Starts

Volume 127: Accepting Life in a Wheelchair
Volume 128: Understanding and Overcoming Homesickness
Volume 129: Understanding and Overcoming Wanderlust
Volume 130: Dizziness, Meniere's Disease
Volume 131: Overcoming Aggression
Volume 132: Cutting and Self-Harm
Volume 133: Hair Pulling, Trichotillomania
Volume 134: Postpartum Depression
Volume 135: For Relatives of Dementia Patients
Volume 136: Self-Harm, Artificial Disorders
Volume 137: Activating Self-Healing Powers
Volume 138: Preventing Depression Relapse
Volume 139: Reactive Psychoses, Follow-Up
Volume 140: Obsessive Thoughts and Impulses
Volume 141: Compulsive Checking
Volume 142: Compulsive Counting, Symmetry Obsession
Volume 143: Compulsive Washing, Cleanliness Obsession
Volume 144: Compulsive Questioning
Volume 145: Dissociative Paralysis
Volume 146: Phantom Pain
Volume 147: Overcoming Complaining
Volume 148: Hay Fever, Pollen Allergy
Volume 149: Sexual Abuse, Victim Support
Volume 150: Standing Strong Against Sexism, #metoo
Volume 151: Binge Eating
Volume 152: Overcoming Thoughts of Revenge
Volume 153: Detachment from the Aggressor, Stockholm Syndrome
Volume 154: Courage to Separate
Volume 155: Chronic Fatigue, Exhaustion
Volume 156: Fear of the Future, Existential Anxiety
Volume 157: Excessive Worry About Children
Volume 158: Fear of Failure

Volume 159: Ending Distrust and Control
Volume 160: Dejection, Dysphoria
Volume 161: Boreout, Chronic Boredom
Volume 162: Bipolar Disorders, Relapse Prevention
Volume 163: Mania, Relapse Prevention
Volume 164: Nihilism, Feelings of Worthlessness
Volume 165: Thumb Sucking
Volume 166: Being Brave
Volume 167: Being Proud
Volume 168: Overcoming Shyness
Volume 169: Being Able to Delegate Responsibility
Volume 170: Being Able to Show Emotions
Volume 171: Letting Go of Guilt, Victim Support
Volume 172: Processing Guilt, Offender Support
Volume 173: Mood Swings, Cyclothymia
Volume 174: Lack of Drive, Vital Sadness
Volume 175: Hearing Voices with Reality Reference
Volume 176: Confident Communication
Volume 177: Standing Up for Oneself
Volume 178: Taking New Paths
Volume 179: Confident Job Application
Volume 180: No Longer Being Taken Advantage Of
Volume 181: End of Submissiveness
Volume 182: Depressive Numbness
Volume 183: Mood Drops, Affective Incontinence
Volume 184: Mood Instability
Volume 185: Somatoform Disorders
Volume 186: Stomach Ulcer, Psychosomatic
Volume 187: Accepting Amputation
Volume 188: Overcoming and Letting Go of Hatred
Volume 189: Ending Accusations
Volume 190: Allowing Tears, Being Able to Cry

Volume 191: Finding and Sorting Repressed Feelings
Volume 192: Somatoform Pain
Volume 193: Living Autonomously
Volume 194: Anhedonia, Joylessness
Volume 195: Persistent Sadness
Volume 196: Obesity, Food Addiction
Volume 197: Parents of Abused Children
Volume 198: Letting Go and Letting Be
Volume 199: Childhood Sexual Abuse
Volume 200: Fear of Loss

www.Ingramcontent.com/pod-product-compliance
Lightning Source LLC
Chambersburg PA
CBHW030459220526
45464CB00006B/2579